THE BEGINNERS BUSINESS GUIDE TO PROFITABLE ALOE VERA FARMING

Harnessing Nature's Gift: Practical Tips for a Successful Aloe Vera Farming Venture

KARAN IRIS

DISCLAIMER

This book's content is only meant to be used for general informative purposes. Although the author has taken great care to ensure the content is accurate and thorough, no warranties or assurances on the information's accuracy, correctness, or reliability are provided. It is recommended that readers employ their own judgment and discretion when applying any material found in this book to their particular situation.

The information in this book is not intended to replace professional advice, nor is the author an expert in any of the subjects covered. It is recommended that readers consult with experienced professionals regarding any particular issues or concerns.

Any name that may be mentioned or referred in this book does not imply endorsement, recommendation, or relationship on the part of the author with any person, entity, good, website, or association. These references are made only for informational purposes and are not meant to be taken as recommendations or endorsements.

The information contained in this book may cause readers to suffer loss or damage, for which the author disclaims all obligation and accountability. The only people accountable for the decisions and actions taken by readers using the information presented are themselves.

Any names, characters, companies, locations, activities, occasions, and incidents referenced in this book are either made up or the result of the author's imagination. Any likeness to real people, living or dead, or to real things is entirely coincidental.

This book's content may change at any time, without prior notice, according to the author. The onus is on the reader to verify whether there have been any updates or revisions.

The reader accepts the conditions of this disclaimer by reading this book. Please do not

read this book or use its contents if you do not
agree to these terms.

Table of Contents

CHAPTER 1...10

OVERVIEW OF ALOE VERA AGRICULTURE

....10

Comprehending Aloe Vera Fundamentals 10

Aloe Vera's Historical and Contemporary Uses

....12

The Aloe Vera Farm's Economic Potential 13

A Synopsis of the Aloe Vera Sector 15

CHAPTER 3 18

BEGINNING 18

The Novice's Handbook for Successful Aloe

Vera Farming 18

Getting the Soil Ready for Growing Aloe Vera20

Finding High-Grade Aloe Vera Plants 21

Configuring Watering Systems........................23

CHAPTER 3 26

ALOE VERA PLANTING 26

The Best Ways to Plant Aloe Vera 26

Planting and Spacing Methods........................27

Preliminary Inspection and Upkeep 29

Typical Errors to Prevent 30

CHAPTER 4 34

GROWTH AND DEVELOPMENT OF ALOE VERA 34

Comprehending the Development Phases 34

Ideal Growing Environments 36

Handling Growth-Related Issues 40

CHAPTER 5 44

HOW TO KEEP UP YOUR ALOE VERA FARM 44

Routine Maintenance Procedures 44

Soil Health and Fertilization 45

Disease Control and Prevention 47

CHAPTER 6 50

HOW TO GATHER ALOE VERA 50

Choosing the Appropriate Time to Harvest 50

Selection Methods 51

Handling and Storing After Harvest 52

Improving Quality and Yield......54

CHAPTER 7 58

ALOE VERA GOODS AND METHODS 58

Products and Processing of Aloe Vera......58

Overview of Products Using Aloe Vera 58

Methods of Processing Aloe Vera Gel and Juice 60

Aloe Vera Value-Added Products 62

Configuring a Unit for Processing 63

CHAPTER 8......68

PROMOTING AND DISTRIBUTING ALOE VERA......68

Determining Target Audiences 68

Formulating a Marketing Plan 70

Establishing Your Aloe Vera Product Brand ...73

Sales Techniques and Distribution Channels .74

CHAPTER 9......80

MANAGING MONEY IN ALOE VERA FARMING......80

Cost-Budgeting and Analysis 80

Strategies for Pricing 82

Handling Farm Funding..................................84

Opportunities for Funding and Investment....86

CHAPTER 10 88

GROWING AND SCALING YOUR ALOE VERA COMPANY 88

Selecting Possibilities for Growth 88

Diversification Techniques: 90

Forging Alliances and Cooperations.........91

Long-Term Growth and Sustainability 93

CHAPTER 1

OVERVIEW OF ALOE VERA AGRICULTURE

Succulent plants like aloe vera, which have therapeutic and cosmetic uses, are becoming more and more well-liked among farmers because of their high economic worth and low maintenance needs. Understanding the needs of the plant's cultivation, consumer demand, and financial potential is essential for profitable aloe vera farming. For those who are new to aloe vera farming, this guide offers a thorough overview that includes information on the industry landscape, history, and economic feasibility of the plant.

Comprehending Aloe Vera Fundamentals

Botanical Features

The Asphodelaceae family includes the perennial xerophytic plant aloe vera. Its thick, meaty leaves are filled with a material that resembles gel and is said to have medicinal qualities. The plant may thrive in areas with little rainfall since it is well-suited to arid and semi-arid conditions.

Requirements for Cultivation

1. **Climate**: Warm, dry regions between 20°C and 30°C (68°F and 86°F) are ideal for aloe vera growth. Both extended wetness and freezing are intolerable to it.

2. **Soil**: The plant likes sandy or loamy soil that drains well and has a pH of 6.0 to 7.5. Root rot can be avoided with proper drainage.

3. **Watering**: Moderate watering is necessary for aloe vera. Root deterioration might result from overwatering, hence it should be avoided. In most cases, watering once every three weeks is adequate.

4. **Sunlight**: Aloe vera grows best in full sun, however it may take little shade. It is advised to get at least 6–8 hours of sunlight each day.

5. **Spacing**: To promote proper air circulation and growth, plants should be placed roughly 60 centimeters (24 inches) apart.

Methods of Propagation

Aloe vera can be multiplied by leaf cuttings, offsets (puppies), or seeds. The most popular and efficient technique for commercial growing is offsets. These tiny plants, which emerge from the mother plant's base, are divided and moved to different areas.

Aloe Vera's Historical and Contemporary Uses

Historical Applications

Many cultures have utilized aloe vera for thousands of years. The "plant of immortality" was known to the ancient Egyptians, who incorporated it into their funeral rites. Greek and Roman doctors also used it to treat wounds and stomach issues.

Contemporary Uses

Aloe vera is widely used in the culinary, pharmaceutical, and cosmetic industries today. Among its uses are:

1. **Cosmetics**: Because of its calming and moisturizing qualities, aloe vera gel is a staple in skin care products like moisturizers, sunscreens, and anti-aging lotions.

2. **Pharmaceuticals**: Topical ointments and lotions containing aloe vera extracts are used to treat burns, wounds, and skin diseases like psoriasis and eczema.

3. **Food and Drinks**: Aloe vera juice and supplements are used for their alleged health benefits, which include bolstering the immune system and enhancing digestion.

The Aloe Vera Farm's Economic Potential

Aloe vera farming is a desirable alternative for farmers because of its numerous economic benefits.

1. **Low Maintenance Costs**: Aloe vera requires very little in the way of inputs like pesticides and fertilizers once it has been established. Because of its drought tolerance, less frequent irrigation is required.

2. Aloe vera plants have a **high yield** and can be picked many times a year. Considerable harvests can be produced by a well-maintained aloe vera farm, guaranteeing a consistent income.

3. **Market Demand**: The demand for products containing aloe vera has increased due to consumers' growing awareness of natural and organic products. It is anticipated that this tendency will continue, giving aloe vera growers a steady market.

4. **Value-Added Products**: By turning aloe vera leaves into juice, gel, or powder, farmers can increase their profits by producing higher-priced, value-added goods.

A Synopsis of the Aloe Vera Sector

Worldwide Market Patterns

The growing customer preference for natural and organic products is fueling the expansion of the aloe vera market globally. Europe, Asia-Pacific, and the United States are important markets. Aloe vera is most commonly used in the beauty and personal care industries, with the food and pharmaceutical sectors following closely behind.

Important Manufacturers and Exporters

The top producers of aloe vera are the United States, Mexico, China, and India. These nations have developed processing infrastructure to satisfy global demand in addition to enjoying advantageous meteorological conditions.

Opportunities and Difficulties

1. **Difficulties**:

- **Climate Sensitivity**: Aloe vera cultivation may be restricted in some areas because of its sensitivity to extreme cold and dampness.

- **Market Competition**: As aloe vera becomes more and more popular, producer competition also increases, which may have an impact on pricing and profitability.

- **Quality Control**: Upholding regulatory requirements and the market's confidence in aloe vera products depend on their constant purity and quality.

2. **Chances**:

Innovative goods: New aloe vera-based goods, like nutraceuticals and functional foods, may be developed.

- **Sustainable agricultural**: Using sustainable agricultural techniques will help you reach specialized markets and draw in environmentally conscientious customers.

- **Study and Development**: Ongoing study into the therapeutic characteristics of aloe vera can lead to new applications and boost its value.

In summary, aloe vera cultivation offers novice farmers a feasible and lucrative agricultural endeavor. Farmers might prosper in this sector by comprehending the requirements of the plant, taking advantage of its traditional and contemporary applications, and capitalizing on the expanding market demand.

CHAPTER 3

BEGINNING

The Novice's Handbook for Successful Aloe Vera Farming

Selecting the Appropriate Site

The success of your aloe vera farming depends on your choice of site. These are the main points to remember:

1. **Climate**: Hot, dry areas are ideal for aloe vera growth. It can withstand high temperatures of up to 40°C (104°F), however it prefers a temperature range of 25–30°C (77–86°F). Because aloe vera is sensitive to cold temperatures and frost can harm or kill the plants, make sure there isn't much frost in the area.

2. Aloe vera requires an abundance of sunlight. Pick a spot that gets six to eight hours of direct sunlight every day. Sunburn can be avoided in

severely hot areas by finding some shade during the warmest portion of the day.

3. **Rainfall**: Aloe vera is drought-tolerant and doesn't need a lot of water. However, root rot can result from excessive rain or inadequate drainage. Seek out an area with 500–800 mm of evenly distributed annual rainfall. Make sure adequate drainage systems are installed if the area experiences increased rainfall.

4. **Soil**: Sandy-loamy soil with adequate drainage is preferred for aloe vera. The ideal pH range for soil is 6.0–7.0, which is neutral to slightly acidic.

 Steer clear of regions with chronic waterlogging or dense clay soils.

5. **Accessibility**: Verify that labor, tools, and the transportation of harvested leaves to markets or processing facilities can all reach the spot. The cost and efficiency of operations can be greatly impacted by a location's proximity to infrastructure and highways.

Getting the Soil Ready for Growing Aloe Vera

It needs proper soil preparation to guarantee strong growth and large yields. Take these actions:

1. **Soil Testing**: Test the soil to find out its pH, texture, and nutritional content. This will assist in determining any imbalances or weaknesses that require correction.

2. **Clearing the Land**: Clear the field of any weeds, trash, or abandoned crops. Weeds can pose a threat to aloe vera, particularly during its early growth stages.

3. **Tilling and Leveling**: To increase aeration and root penetration, till the soil down to a depth of roughly 30 cm. To guarantee even water distribution and avoid waterlogging, level the terrain.

4. **Amending the Soil**: To increase fertility and drainage, amend the soil with organic matter, such as compost or well-rotted manure, based on

the findings of the soil test. Thoroughly mix these amendments into the soil.

5. **Building Raised Beds**: To improve drainage and avoid water stagnation around the roots, build raised beds or ridges in places that are prone to high rainfall or poor drainage.

6. **Mulching**: After planting, surround the plants with a layer of mulch, such as straw or organic leftovers. Mulching aids in controlling temperature, weed suppression, and moisture retention.

Finding High-Grade Aloe Vera Plants

The output and financial success of your farm are directly impacted by the caliber of your aloe vera plants. Here's where to find premium plants:

1. **Variety Selection**: Select an aloe vera variety that is appropriate for your climate and soil type. Because of its high gel content and therapeutic qualities, Aloe barbadensis miller is

the most widely used and commercially viable cultivar.

2. **Reputable Suppliers**: Purchase your plants from suppliers or nurseries who have a solid reputation for offering premium, disease-free planting material. To avoid bringing pests or illnesses to your farm, steer clear of purchasing from dubious sources.

3. **Healthy Plants**: Choose plants that are robust, disease-free, and devoid of visible pests. Seek for plants that have four or more fully grown leaves and well-developed roots.

4. **Propagation Methods**: Tissue culture, offsets (puppies), and seeds can all be used to multiply aloe vera. The most popular technique for commercial growing is offsets because they guarantee faster establishment and genetic consistency.

5. **Transport and Handling**: To prevent damage, make sure the plants are handled and transported properly. To lessen transplant shock, keep the roots moist while being transported and plant them as soon as possible.

Configuring Watering Systems

Growing aloe vera successfully requires effective irrigation, particularly in areas with erratic rainfall. How to Install a Successful Irrigation System:

1. **Water Needs**: Aloe vera doesn't need a lot of water. Rotten roots can result from over-irrigation. When plants are generating offsets, right after planting, and during dry spells are the crucial times for irrigation.

2. **Watering Techniques**:

- **Drip Irrigation**: This is the most effective technique because it minimizes runoff and evaporation by supplying water straight to the root zone of the plant. It aids in preserving ideal soil moisture content.

- **Sprinkler irrigation**: This works well for bigger fields, but watch out for how soon the foliage dries to avoid fungal diseases.

- **Manual Irrigation**: Although labor-intensive, manual irrigation using hoses or watering cans can be enough for small-scale farms.

3. **Water Quality**: For irrigation, use clear, non-saline water. Plant growth and gel quality might be impacted by high salinity.

4. **Scheduling**: To minimize evaporation losses, water the plants either early in the morning or late at night. The type of soil, climate, and stage of plant growth all affect how often and how much watering is needed.

5. **Maintenance**: Make sure the irrigation system is regularly inspected and maintained to avoid leaks, blockage, and other problems that could compromise the distribution of water.

You can start a successful, productive, and sustainable aloe vera farm by carefully weighing these factors.

CHAPTER 3

ALOE VERA PLANTING

The Best Ways to Plant Aloe Vera

Although aloe vera is a hardy plant that can survive in a variety of environments, following recommended practices guarantees healthy growth and a successful harvest. Here's a comprehensive guide to effectively planting aloe vera:

1. **Soil and Climate Requirements:**

Climate: Warm, dry areas are ideal for aloe vera growth. Being a succulent, it can withstand severe droughts because its leaves retain water. The range of ideal temperatures is 13°C to 27°C (55°F to 80°F).

- **Soil:** To avoid root rot, aloe vera needs soil that drains well. The best soils are loamy or sandy, with a pH of 6.0 to 8.0. Steer clear of clayey soils or improve drainage by adding gravel or sand.

2. **Selection of Site:**

- Pick a bright area with plenty of ventilation. Every day, aloe vera plants require six to eight hours of direct sunlight.

Make sure the location is, if at all possible, somewhat raised to aid with water runoff.

3. **Season of Planting:**

- When the weather is warmer, plant aloe vera in the spring or early summer. By doing this, the plant can develop roots before it encounters colder weather.

Planting and Spacing Methods

Proper spacing and planting practices are vital for healthy Aloe Vera plants and optimum yield:

1. **Distance:**

- Leave a minimum of 18 to 24 inches (45 to 60 cm) between each plant. This gap gives each plant adequate room to grow and spread out without having to compete with one another for resources.

It is recommended that rows be placed 24 to 36 inches (60 to 90 cm) apart to provide easy maintenance and air circulation.

2. **Tips for Planting:**

Propagation: Offsets, or pups, are the usual means of spreading aloe vera. These are little clones that encircle the mature plant's root.

Set Up: Make sure the pups have some roots connected before carefully removing them from the parent plant. To avoid rot, let the offsets dry for a few days before planting.

- **Planting:** Before planting, dig a hole that is deep enough to bury the roots but not the foliage. To secure the plant, place the offset in the hole, cover it with soil, and gently press down. First, use water cautiously to prevent waterlogging.

Preliminary Inspection and Upkeep

The growth and productivity of Aloe Vera plants depend heavily on the initial and continuous care they receive:

1. **Sprinkling:**

- Use minimal water to the plants. Aloe vera thrives in dry environments and can withstand droughts. Rotten roots might result from overwatering.

- Water sparingly in the initial weeks following planting to aid with root establishment. After the soil is established, water it deeply but sparingly, letting it dry out in between applications.

2. **Conception:**

- Heavy fertilizing is not necessary for aloe vera plants. To promote growth, apply a balanced, diluted fertilizer (10-40-10) once a year in the spring.

Prevent overfertilization as it may cause damage to the plant.

3. **Sweating:**

Cover the plants with a thin layer of organic mulch to help them retain moisture and keep weeds at bay. To avoid rot, make sure the mulch stays away from the plant's roots.

4. **Disease and Pest Management:**

Though largely pest-free, aloe vera occasionally becomes infected with fungi, mealybugs, or aphids.

- Regularly check plants, and use neem oil or insecticidal soap to cure pests. Make sure there is enough airflow to stop the growth of fungi.

Typical Errors to Prevent

Aloe Vera plant health and yield can be greatly enhanced by avoiding typical pitfalls:

1. **Over-saturation:**

- Overwatering is among the most frequent errors. Very little water is needed for aloe vera. Make sure the soil dries out entirely in between applications of water.

2. **Inadequate Drainage:**

- Root rot can result from planting in soil that holds too much water. Avoid heavy, clayey soils and choose well-draining soil instead.

3. **Inadequate Natural Light:**

Aloe Vera plants need lots of sunlight to thrive. If you plant them in shaded regions, their growth may become weak and lanky. Make sure they get six to eight hours of direct sunlight every day.

4. **Overcrowding:**

- Planting aloe vera too near to one another might result in poor air circulation and competition for resources, which raises the risk of illness. Respect the advised distance guidelines.

5. **Ignoring pH of Soil:**

- Aloe vera favors soil that is slightly acidic above neutral. To keep the pH of the soil within the ideal range of 6.0 to 8.0, test it frequently and amend it as needed.

You may guarantee a productive and healthy aloe vera farm by adhering to these best practices, planting methods, and maintenance advice as well as avoiding typical blunders.

CHAPTER 4

GROWTH AND DEVELOPMENT OF ALOE VERA

The Novice's Handbook for Successful Aloe Vera Farming

If done properly, aloe vera farming may be a very profitable endeavor. This comprehensive book will help you grasp every important facet of aloe vera growth and development.

Comprehending the Development Phases

Aloe vera plants go through several growth phases, and to ensure healthy development and optimize yield, each stage requires specialized care and maintenance.

1. **Stage of Germination**:

Stay: two to four weeks.

Details: When given enough moisture, warmth, and light, seeds will sprout. Since it establishes the framework for plant health, this stage is crucial.

- **Treatment**: Keep the soil moist but not soggy, and make sure it's between 20 and 25°C. To prevent root rot, use a soil mixture that drains effectively.

2. **Seedling Phase**:

Size: two to three months.

- **Details**: As seedlings sprout, they start to form their first real leaves. The plant grows slowly during this stage as it establishes its root system.

- **Treatment**: Offer regular moisture, shield from direct sunshine, and shield from inclement weather. Aim for appropriate space to prevent crowding.

3. **Early Stage**:

Duration: One to two years.

- **Details**: The plant develops thicker roots and more robust leaves. The growth rate sharply accelerates.

- **Care**: Use organic compost to maintain soil fertility, gradually increase exposure to direct sunshine, and keep an eye out for pests.

4. **Developed Stage**:

- **Duration**: up to four years.

- **Details**: The plant achieves its full size and starts to generate offsets (pups) that can be utilized for propagation.

- **Care**: Make sure the environment is ideal for growth, harvest leaves frequently to stimulate new growth, and control offsets to maintain output.

Ideal Growing Environments

Creating the proper atmosphere for Aloe Vera is crucial to successful production. Here are some things to think about:

1. **Temperature**:

Temperature: The ideal temperature range for aloe vera is between 20 and 30°C. It has to be protected from frost but can withstand hotter temperatures.

- **Sunlight**: It is best to get 6–8 hours a day of full sun exposure. On the other hand, partial shade is advantageous during peak hours in severely hot climes.

2. **Soil**:

- **Type**: Loamy or sandy soil with good drainage is preferred. Soils with a lot of clay should not be worked since they hold too much water.

- **pH Level**: Soils with a pH of 6.0–7.0 are slightly acidic, which is preferred by aloe vera.

3. **Watering**:

- **Frequency**: Deeply but sporadically water. In between waterings, let the soil dry out.

- **Method**: To stop leaf rot, don't water from above. Water near the plant's base.

4. **Conception**:

- **Type**: Apply a half-strength solution of a balanced, water-soluble fertilizer. Organic compost is also advantageous.

- **Frequency**: During the growing season, fertilize once every two to three months.

Tracking the Health of Plants

High yields and the maintenance of healthy aloe vera plants depend on routine monitoring.

1. **Examining Visually**:

- **Leaves**: Look for lesions, stains, or discoloration that could point to a disease or pest problem.

- **Roots**: Check for pests or rot, particularly if plants exhibit symptoms of stress.

2. **Trends in Growth**:

- **Normal Growth**: Robust, meaty leaves and steady growth are signs of a healthy aloe vera plant.

- **Abnormal development**: Leaf loss, withering, or stunted development may be signs of underlying issues.

3. **Impact and Illness Control**:

- **Common Pests**: Spider mites, mealybugs, and aphids are common culprits. Use insecticidal soap or neem oil as a natural treatment.

- **Diseases**: Ensuring enough drainage and avoiding overwatering will help prevent fungal illnesses like root rot.

4. **Levels of Nutrients**:

- **Symptoms of Deficiency**: Browning tips may indicate a potassium deficiency, whereas yellowing leaves may indicate a nitrogen deficiency.

- **Soil Testing**: Conduct regular soil tests to determine pH balance and nutrient levels. Adapt fertilization as necessary.

Handling Growth-Related Issues

Aloe vera growth will inevitably involve challenges, but many problems can be avoided with proactive management.

1. **Stress in the Environment**:

- **Heat Stress**: To avoid sunburn during periods of intense heat, provide shade.

- **Cold Stress**: During cold snaps, bring potted plants indoors or cover them with frost cloths.

2. **Infestations of Pests**:

- **Identification**: Observe plants frequently for early indications of insect activity.

- **Control Measures**: To manage infestations, use organic insecticides, physical removal, or natural predators.

3. **Illness Control**:

- **Prevention**: To prevent fungal diseases, use sterilized soil and refrain from overwatering.

- **Treatment**: To stop the spread, remove and destroy any afflicted plant parts. Fungicides should only be used last.

4. **Management of Nutrients**:

- **deficits**: Use the right fertilizers to address nutritional deficits as soon as possible.

Toxicities: Steer clear of overfertilization, since this may result in signs of toxicity and nutrient burn.

5. Propagation Problems:

Inadequate Offset Production: Make sure established plants have enough light and are not packed too closely together.

- **Transplanting Stress**: To lessen shock, minimize root disturbance, and provide enough water after transplanting.

Beginners can maximize their aloe vera farming operations and guarantee a lucrative venture by comprehending and addressing these elements. Success requires quick actions, proper care, and routine monitoring.

CHAPTER 5

HOW TO KEEP UP YOUR ALOE VERA FARM

Routine Maintenance Procedures

Watering

Even though aloe vera is resistant to drought, it still requires enough hydration to be healthy. The main goal is to prevent root rot by not overwatering. Give the plants deep, sparing watering, letting the soil dry between applications. Watering your plants once every three weeks should be plenty. Adapt the frequency to the soil type and climate where you live.

Pruning

Pruning aids in keeping aloe vera plants attractive and healthy. Eliminate any infected, dead, or damaged leaves right away. This promotes new development and stops the spread of illnesses and pests. To minimize damage to the plant, make clean cuts with sharp, clean equipment.

Mulching

Mulch is applied to the soil around aloe vera plants to assist control of temperature, weed growth, and soil moisture retention. Make use of organic mulches such as bark, leaves, or straw. To avoid rot, make sure the mulch is not too near the base of the plant.

Soil Health and Fertilization
Soil Conditions

Aloe vera grows best on sandy or loamy soil that drains well and has a pH of 6.0 to 7. 0 is neutral to mildly acidic.

To avoid root rot and waterlogging, proper drainage is essential. To increase drainage, if your soil is mostly clay, you might want to amend it with sand or perlite.

The process of fertilization

Heavy fertilization is not necessary for aloe vera. Healthy development can be encouraged, nevertheless, by applying a balanced, water-soluble fertilizer (10-40-10 NPK) once a year throughout the growing season. Steer clear of high-nitrogen fertilizers since they may result in floppy, mushy leaves. Organic fertilizers and compost are great choices since they improve soil health and release nutrients gradually.

Soil Examination

Frequent soil testing ensures ideal growing conditions by keeping an eye on pH and nutrient levels. Testing should be done every two to three years. Based on the results, amend the soil with the required nutrients or lime to regulate pH.

Pest and Weed Management

Weed Management

Aloe vera faces competition from weeds for light, water, and nutrients. It takes regular weeding to keep plants healthy. Mulch helps keep weeds under control. When weeds do emerge, pull them out right away using a hoe or by hand. Use organic herbicides or landscaping fabric on larger farms.

Termite Management

Although aloe vera is largely pest-free, typical pests like mealybugs, aphids, and spider mites can still cause problems for it. Check plants frequently for indications of infestation. Utilize native predators such as ladybugs to achieve biological control. Use neem oil or insecticidal soaps in cases of severe infestations, but make sure to follow the manufacturer's directions to prevent harming the plants.

Disease Control and Prevention

Typical Illnesses

Diseases include aloe rust, bacterial soft rot, and fungal infections can affect aloe vera. To stop infections from spreading and causing serious harm, early detection and treatment are essential.

Disease Prophylaxis

1. ** Appropriate Spacing**: To enhance air circulation and lower humidity, which aids in preventing bacterial and fungal growth, make sure there is enough space between plants.

2. **Sanitation**: Maintain the growing space hygienic. As soon as possible, remove and discard any sick plant material. To stop infections from spreading, sterilize instruments regularly.

3. **Watering Practices**: Water the base of the plants rather than the leaves to prevent fungal diseases. Steer clear of overhead irrigation, particularly in the late afternoon or evening.

4. **Soil Health**: Keep your soil in good condition by managing pH levels and fertilizing

appropriately. Plants in good health are more disease-resistant.

Infection Control

1. **Monitoring**: Keep an eye out for disease symptoms in plants, such as spots, discoloration, or wilting.

2. **Organic Treatments**: To treat fungal infections, apply organic fungicides such as neem oil or treatments based on copper.

3. **Chemical Treatments**: Chemical fungicides or bactericides may be required in extreme situations. Utilize them as a final option while adhering to all safety precautions to reduce your influence on the environment.

Following these upkeep guidelines will help you maintain a robust, fruitful aloe vera farm that maximizes productivity and quality. The secret to successful aloe vera farming is maintaining ideal growing conditions, implementing the right treatments, and conducting routine monitoring.

CHAPTER 6

HOW TO GATHER ALOE VERA

Choosing the Appropriate Time to Harvest

**1. The plant's maturity: **

- After 18 to 24 months of growth, aloe vera plants usually attain maturity and are suitable for harvesting. The leaves will be thick, meaty, and gel-filled at this point.

- Younger, inner leaves should be allowed to flourish whereas mature leaves are typically found on the outer layers of the plant.

**2. Seasonal Aspects: **

- Aloe Vera can be gathered all year round, although adverse weather should be avoided. To avoid causing heat stress to the plants, it is best to harvest in the cooler hours of the day, such as early morning or late afternoon.

**3. Visual Cues: **

- The leaves have to be at least 12 inches long, firm, and vivid green. Steer clear of picking leaves that are thinning, yellowing, or exhibiting symptoms of illness.

Selection Methods

**1. Instruments and apparatus: **

- To make clean cuts in the leaves, use pruning shears or a sharp knife. This guarantees a clean cut that will mend rapidly and helps shield the plant from harm.

- Use alcohol to clean tools both before and after use to stop contamination and disease transmission.

**2. Method of Cutting: **

Make sure to leave enough interior leaves for the plant to continue growing when choosing the outermost mature leaves.

Trim leaves at the base, keeping them as close to the main stem as you can to avoid damaging the center of the plant.

- To enable adequate sap drainage and quicker wound healing, make a neat, angled cut.

3. Harvest Frequency:

- Harvesting should occur regularly every 6 to 8 weeks, depending on the health and development rate of the plant.

Steer clear of overharvesting from a single plant to maintain its productivity and vigor over time.

Handling and Storing After Harvest

**1. Quick Processing: **

- Rinse the leaves with water after harvesting to get rid of any dirt or debris.

- To avoid sunburn and moisture loss, let the leaves drain and air dry in a shady spot.

**2. Gel Removal: **

- To extract the gel, cut the leaves lengthwise and use a spoon or a gel extractor tool to scoop out the inner gel.

To preserve the gel's quality and purity, make sure that the extraction process is conducted in a clean, hygienic environment.

**3. Conditions of Storage: **

- Fresh aloe vera gel is kept for up to a week in the refrigerator when kept in airtight containers.

- The gel can be dried, frozen, or stabilized by processing it with preservatives for extended storage.

**4. Storage of leaves: **

- Whole leaves can be kept in the refrigerator for up to two weeks when wrapped in plastic wrap or placed in zip-lock bags.

- To avoid rotting, keep the leaves out of direct sunshine and too much moisture.

Improving Quality and Yield

1. Management of Plant Health:

- Continually check plants for illnesses and pests. Use integrated pest management (IPM) techniques to reduce the usage of chemicals and uphold organic standards.

Make careful to water your plants appropriately, preventing waterlogging and encouraging soil that drains effectively.

**2. **Nutrient Management

- To preserve soil fertility and encourage strong development, apply compost or organic fertilizers.

- Identification of nutrient deficits and subsequent modification of fertilization techniques can be facilitated by routine soil testing.

**3. Ideal Conditions for Growth: **

- Aloe Vera grows best in sandy or loamy soil that drains well and has a pH between 6.0 and 7.5.

- Make sure plants get enough sunlight (6–8 hours per day in direct sunlight), and shield them from harsh cold and frost.

**4. Time of Harvest: **

- Harvest leaves in the spring and fall, when conditions are ideal to minimize plant stress and enhance gel quality: early morning or late afternoon.

- To maintain plant health and continual production, implement a rotational harvesting system.

**5. Control of Quality: **

- To maintain high standards, strictly enforce quality control procedures during harvesting, processing, and storage.

- Consistently instruct employees on proper handling techniques for aloe vera to avoid contamination and guarantee product quality.

Beginners may efficiently manage their aloe vera farming operations and guarantee good yield, quality, and profitability according to these instructions.

CHAPTER 7

ALOE VERA GOODS AND METHODS

Products and Processing of Aloe Vera

Aloe Vera is well known for its many health advantages and a broad range of uses in the food and beverage, pharmaceutical, and cosmetic industries. Profitable aloe vera farming requires an understanding of the various products obtained from the plant, the processing methods involved, and how to set up a processing unit. A thorough guide on these topics can be found below.

Overview of Products Using Aloe Vera

**1. Aloe Vera Gel: **

The most well-known Aloe Vera product is the gel, which is made from the parenchyma of the inner leaf. Because of its calming, hydrating, and restorative qualities, it is frequently included in skincare and cosmetic products.

**2. Aloe Vera Juice: **

This is made from aloe vera gel and is meant to be drunk as a healthy beverage. Its benefits for digestion and detoxification are well established.

**3. Powdered Aloe Vera: **

The Aloe Vera gel is prepared by crushing and dehydrating it. It is a component of many goods, such as cosmetics and dietary supplements.

**4. Extracts from Aloe Vera: **

These are concentrated aloe vera extracts made via a variety of extraction techniques. Both nutraceuticals and medications employ them.

**5. Aloe Vera Extract: **

Because of its moisturizing and anti-inflammatory qualities, infused aloe vera oil is utilized in massage oils and hair care products.

**6. Aloe Vera Tablets/Capsules: **

These are nutritional supplements, touted for their health advantages, manufactured from powdered or extracted aloe vera.

Methods of Processing Aloe Vera Gel and Juice

**1. Gathering and Getting Ready:

- Cut mature aloe vera leaves near the root to harvest them.

- Thoroughly wash the leaves to get rid of any dirt or contaminants.

**2. Gel Extraction: **

- Fillet the leaves to reveal the inner gel by removing the outer rind.

- Scoop out the gel using a clean knife or specialist equipment.

**3. Consistency: **

Aloe Vera gel needs to be stabilized right away because it oxidizes easily.

- Refrigeration and the addition of ascorbic or citric acid are common techniques.

**4. Filtration: **

- Filter the gel to get rid of any last bits of solid matter.

Mesh filters or specialized filtration apparatus can be used for this.

5. ** Pasteurization:

- Heat the gel so that any microbiological impurities are eliminated without affecting the bioactive ingredients.

- The gel is usually heated for a brief period to 65–70°C.

6. Manufacturing of Aloe Vera Juice:

- To prepare juice, blend the stabilized gel with water.

Preservatives and flavorings are examples of additional substances that can be added.

**7. Packaging and Bottling: **

Verify that every container and piece of equipment has been sterilized.

- Pour aloe vera juice or gel into the bottles, then seal them right away.

Aloe Vera Value-Added Products

**1. Products for Skincare: **

- Aloe Vera is used in creams, lotions, and gels because of its healing and moisturizing qualities.

**2. Products for Haircare: **

- Aloe Vera-based shampoos and conditioners that condition hair and support healthy scalps.

**3. Nutritional Supplements: **

- Aloe Vera powders, tablets, and capsules touted for their immune-stimulating and digestive properties.

**4. Drinks: **

- Aloe Vera drinks and smoothies, provide a hydrating and nutritious beverage choice.

**5. Pharmaceuticals: **

- Aloe Vera extracts are utilized for their medicinal properties in oral formulations and topical ointments.

**6. Cosmetics: **

- Aloe Vera is used in makeup products, like primers and foundation, because of its calming effects.

Configuring a Unit for Processing

**1. Infrastructure and Location: **

- To cut down on travel time, pick a site close to aloe vera plantations.

- Verify that the facility has enough room for storage, packing, and processing.

**2. Tools: **

- Pasteurizers, blenders, filling and sealing machines, filtration units, washing tanks, and sterilizing equipment are examples of essential equipment.

- Make a quality equipment investment to guarantee effective processing and superior product quality.

**3. Control of Quality: **

- Put strict quality control procedures in place to guarantee the effectiveness and purity of aloe vera products.

- Conduct routine tests for the presence of bioactive compounds, chemical stability, and microbiological contamination.

4. Adherence to Regulation:

- Comply with national and international laws governing food and cosmetics.

- Obtain certifications that are required, such as ISO and Good Manufacturing Practices (GMP) certificates.

**5. Employee Education: **

- Teach employees the right handling and processing methods to preserve the integrity of the product.

- Verify their familiarity with quality control and hygiene protocols.

**6. Promotion and Dissemination:

- Create a strong marketing plan to advertise Aloe Vera goods.

- Create avenues of distribution, such as websites, physical stores, and alliances with other companies.

Understanding the wide range of goods that may be made from aloe vera, learning the processing methods to preserve product quality, developing value-added products, and setting up a well-equipped processing facility are all necessary for starting a profitable aloe vera processing business. Aloe Vera cultivation may be made profitable and sustainable with a strategic strategy that makes use of the plant's well-known health advantages and broad popularity.

CHAPTER 8

PROMOTING AND DISTRIBUTING ALOE VERA

Determining Target Audiences

Aware of Your Product:

- **Product Types:** Aloe Vera juice, gel, raw leaves, cosmetics, and health supplements.

- **Product Benefits:** Skincare (moisturizing, anti-inflammatory), hair care (nourishing, anti-dandruff), and health benefits (digestive health, immunological support).

Determining Possible Clients:

- **Demographics:** Gender, age, income bracket, and location.

- **Healthy people:** Prefer natural cures and dietary supplements.

- **Skincare and beauty enthusiasts:** Look for natural and organic skincare and cosmetics.

Active lifestyle enthusiasts: Interested in detox beverages and health supplements.

- **Environmentalists:** Prefer environmentally friendly and sustainable goods.

Psychographics: Interests, values, and way of life.

- **Proponents of natural living:** Give preference to chemical-free, organic items.

- **Wellness community:** Groups that promote holistic wellness and health.

Division of the Market:

Regional preferences and urban vs rural areas are divided under **Geographic Segmentation**.

- **Demographic Segmentation:** Income brackets, age categories (millennials, Gen X, baby boomers).

- **Behavioral Segmentation:** Purchase patterns, loyalty status, and usage volume (heavy vs. light users).

Market Analysis:

- **Competitor Analysis:** Determine the main competitors' offerings, costs, and market share.

- **Customer Surveys and Feedback:** Recognize the wants, needs, and pain areas of your customers.

- **Industry Trends:** Keep abreast of developments in emerging markets, consumer behavior, and the market.

Formulating a Marketing Plan

Determining Goals:

- **Short-term Objectives:** Raise initial sales, create leads, and raise brand recognition.

- **Long-term Objectives:** Develop a strong consumer base, create a market presence and experience consistent growth.

Structure of Product:

- **Unique Selling Proposition (USP)**: Emphasize the distinctive qualities of your aloe vera products, such as their organic origin, local sourcing, and exceptional quality.

- **Brand Messaging:** Create a message that appeals to your target audience and is both clear and appealing.

**Marketing Mix: The Four Ps

- **Product:** Guarantee superior quality, efficient packaging, and a wide selection of products.

Price: Competitive pricing approach; take loyalty plans and discounts into account.

- **Place:** Pick the appropriate channels for distribution (online retailers, physical stores, health stores).

- **Promotion:** Make use of a range of promotional instruments (influencer relationships, email marketing, social media).

Online Advertising:

- **Website Optimization:** A visually stunning, educational, and user-friendly website.

Content Marketing: Infographics, films, and blogs describing the uses and advantages of aloe vera.

- **SEO and SEM:** Boost visibility with targeted ads and search engine ranking.

- **Social Media Marketing:** Consistent participation on Facebook, Instagram, and Twitter.

Offline Promotion:

- **Events and Trade Shows:** Attend beauty expos and health and wellness fairs.

Advertisements in local newspapers and health magazines are examples of print media.

- **Networking:** Establish connections with distributors, retailers, and business leaders.

Establishing Your Aloe Vera Product Brand

Identity of Brand:

- **Logo and Design:** Produce a distinctive logo and dependable design components.

- **Brand Colors and Fonts:** Select hues and fonts that capture the essence of your brand.

History of the Brand:

- **Origin Story:** Describe the history and purpose of your company.

- **Core Values:** Emphasize principles like excellence, sustainability, and client happiness.

Voice of Brand:

- **Tone and Style:** Choose an agreeable, formal, and authoritative tone for all of your communications.

- **Consistency:** Make sure that all marketing materials and platforms are consistent.

Interaction with Customers:

- **Social Media Interaction:** Use messages, comments, and interactive material to interact with your fans.

- **Customer Service:** Respond quickly to questions and concerns while offering exceptional customer service.

Reputation Trust:

- **Transparency:** Be open and honest about the sourcing, production, and ingredient lists of your products.

- **Testimonials and Reviews:** Promote and highlight client endorsements and success tales.

Certifications: To establish credibility, obtain certifications (such as organic and cruelty-free).

Sales Techniques and Distribution Channels

Channels of Distribution:

- **Direct Sales:**

-   **Online shopping:** Personal website, Amazon, eBay.

- **Social Media Stores:** Shop for Instagram and Facebook.

- **Sales at Retail:**

Health Stores: Collaborate with national and local health food retailers.

- **Beauty Stores:** Stock skincare and beauty products in physical stores.

- **Supermarkets:** Guaranteed shelf space at food stores and supermarkets.

Wholesale:

Collaborate with distributors to expand your market reach.

- **Bulk Sales:** Provide spas, salons, and wellness centers with bulk purchases.

Marketing Techniques:

- **Individual Sales:**

- **Sales Representatives:** Use competent sales representatives to advertise products.

- **Product Demonstrations:** Give away free samples and show off your products at events and retail locations.

- **Online Sales:**

- **Affiliate Marketing:** Collaborate with influencers and bloggers to market goods.

- **Email marketing:** Create an email list and distribute promos and newsletters regularly.

Discounts and Promotions:

- **Seasonal Sales:** Provide reductions on holidays and other noteworthy events.

- **Loyalty Programs:** Reward loyal consumers with loyalty programs.

Upselling and Bundling:

- **Product Bundles:** Provide lower prices for combined products.

-   **Upsell:** Make complimentary product suggestions at the point of sale.

Materials:

- **Supply Chain Management:** Guarantee a consistent flow of raw materials and prompt manufacturing.

- **Inventory Management:** Monitor demand and stock levels via inventory management systems.

-   **Shipping and Delivery:** Assist reputable shipping firms to ensure timely delivery.

Tracking Performance:

- **Sales Analytics:** Track sales information to spot patterns and gauge progress.

-   **Customer Feedback:** Get input to make goods and services better.

- **Market Adaptation:** Adjust tactics in response to shifting consumer demands and market conditions. Be adaptable.

You may effectively market and sell aloe vera goods and ensure a prosperous and sustainable farming business by comprehending and putting these principles into practice.

CHAPTER 9

MANAGING MONEY IN ALOE VERA FARMING

Cost-Budgeting and Analysis

**1. Setup Fees at First: **

- **Land Acquisition or Lease:** Prices vary according to the land's size, location, and condition.

- **Soil Preparation:** Consists of soil testing, leveling, and plowing. The best soil health may necessitate the use of organic amendments.

- **Seedlings/Plants:** Get premium aloe vera plants or seedlings. Prices differ according to provider and variety.

- **Irrigation System:** Invest in an appropriate irrigation system (since drip irrigation uses less water, it is frequently recommended for aloe vera).

- **Security and Fencing:** Keep animals, vermin, and unwanted access away from your farm.

**2. Regular Operating Expenses: **

Pay for planting, upkeep, harvesting, and processing labor.

- **Pesticides and Fertilizers:** Chemical or organic inputs to guarantee wholesome plant growth.

- **Electricity and Water:** The price of maintaining irrigation systems and other machinery.

- **Maintenance:** Consistent upkeep of infrastructure and equipment.

**3. Extra Fees: **

- **Packaging and Processing:** The price of washing, chopping, and packing aloe vera goods.

Transportation: Delivering products to warehouses or marketplaces.

Sales and Marketing: Advertising costs associated with product promotion.

**4. Setting a budget: **

- **Estimate Revenues and Expenses:** To calculate profitability, project your sales revenue and total estimated costs.

- **Contingency Funds:** Set aside money for emergencies or unanticipated costs.

Financial Planning: Create both short- and long-term financial plans to direct your business's expansion and operations.

Strategies for Pricing

**1. Price-Plus Structure: **

Compute the production's overall cost.

Include a markup to guarantee a profit. This markup ought to yield a return on investment and cover operating expenses.

**2. Competitive Rates: **

Examine the prices of competitors.

- Establish pricing by market norms, but make sure that your special selling point (such as greater quality or organic certification) supports your price.

**3. Value-Added Pricing:

Set the price of your aloe vera goods according to what the consumer thinks they are worth.

- Take into account elements like exclusivity, organic status, and health advantages.

**4. Dynamic Pricing: **

- Modify prices by supply and demand.

- Offer special prices during times of low supply or strong demand, or discounts during times of high supply.

**5. Pricing for Penetration: **

- Lower pricing at first to get into the market and draw clients.

- As your brand becomes more well-known and recognizable to consumers, progressively raise prices.

Handling Farm Funding

1. Maintaining Financial Records:

- Keep thorough records of every transaction, including earnings, outlays, and investments.

- For precise and effective financial management, use accounting software or work with a professional accountant.

2. Management of Cash Flow:

- Keep an eye on your cash flow to make sure you have enough to pay for running expenses.

- Budget for changes in income and expenses with the seasons.

**3. Forecasting and Budgeting: **

- Create quarterly, yearly, and monthly budgets.

- Project future financial success by analyzing market patterns and previous data.

**4. Cost Management: **

Determine where expenses might be cut without sacrificing quality.

Adopt cost-cutting strategies include resource optimization, energy-efficient procedures, and bulk purchasing.

**5. Analysis of Finances: **

Examine financial statements regularly to determine solvency, liquidity, and profitability.

- Assess performance and make wise decisions by using financial ratios and metrics.

Opportunities for Funding and Investment

**1. Individual Reserves: **

- Pay for initial setup and running expenditures out of your savings. This is frequently the least risky and easiest choice.

**2. Loans from banks: **

- Apply for agricultural loans from banks. To obtain money, create a strong business strategy and financial predictions.

- Recognize the conditions, interest rates, and payback schedules.

**3. Federal Awards & Subsidies:

- Look into government initiatives that provide low-interest loans, grants, or subsidies for projects related to agriculture.

- Remain up to date on application procedures and eligibility requirements.

**4. Individual Investors:

- Draw in private investors by demonstrating the aloe vera farm's potential for sustainability and profitability.

- As stipulated in the investment agreement, be ready to split profits or equity.

**5. Using crowdfunding: **

- Start a crowdfunding campaign, usually on internet sites, to collect money from a large number of donors.

- Provide rewards or incentives to entice supporters.

**6. Farmers' Associations: **

- Join or start cooperatives to access chances for group funding and to combine resources.

- Cooperatives might offer extra assistance with marketing and large purchases.

CHAPTER 10

GROWING AND SCALING YOUR ALOE VERA COMPANY

Selecting Possibilities for Growth

Before growing your aloe vera business, it's important to thoroughly assess the opportunities that are present. This entails determining possible growth opportunities, comprehending customer preferences, and evaluating market demand. Here are some things to consider doing:

1. Market Research: To determine the local, national, and international demand for aloe vera products, conduct thorough market research. Examine market trends, customer behavior, and aloe vera industry competition.

2. SWOT Analysis: Evaluate your present business operations by identifying your SWOT factors (Strengths, Weaknesses, Opportunities, and Threats). Determine your company's

prospects for growth, vulnerabilities that need to be fixed, strengths that may be used to your advantage, and possible dangers.

3. Financial Analysis: Assess if expanding would be financially feasible. Determine the expenses related to increasing production, marketing, distribution, and other company facets. Estimated profits and possible returns on investment.

4. Evaluating Infrastructure: Examine your present infrastructure, which includes distribution networks, manufacturing sites, and supply chain coordination. Assess the need for expansions or upgrades to accommodate higher production and escalating demand.

5. Regulatory Compliance: Make sure that the cultivation and production of aloe vera products comply with all applicable laws and industry regulations. Recognize any obstacles—legal or regulatory—that could affect your goals for growth.

You may decide on the best course of action for growing your aloe vera business by carefully weighing these factors.

Diversification Techniques:

In the aloe vera industry, diversification is essential for reducing risks and increasing income sources. Consider the following diversification tactics:

1. Product Diversification: Increase the variety of goods you offer by introducing aloe vera-based juices, gels, cosmetics, supplements, and other items. Reaching out to diverse market sectors can facilitate the acquisition of new clientele.

2. Diversify your product line by looking into additional geographic markets for your aloe vera offerings. Think about focusing on specialized markets inside your current market or selling to overseas areas.

3. Vertical Integration: If you're thinking about growing into upstream or downstream operations, think about vertical integration.

Possessing retail stores, processing plants, or aloe vera plantations could help you gain control over the supply chain and increase your profit margin.

4. Value-Added Services: Provide value-added services to target industries like healthcare, beauty, or agriculture, such as consultancy, training, or specialized aloe vera solutions.

5. Sustainability Initiatives: Apply eco-friendly packaging, organic certifications, or the promotion of moral agricultural methods to include sustainability in your diversification plan.

You can lessen your reliance on a particular product or market and generate potential for long-term success by diversifying your firm.

Forging Alliances and Cooperations

Developing alliances and working together is essential to growing your aloe vera business. Here's how to deal with them successfully:

1. Supplier Partnerships: Form alliances with dependable vendors for equipment, raw materials, and aloe vera plants. To uphold product standards, make sure sourcing is consistent and quality controlled.

2. Distribution Partnerships: To increase your market reach, work with retailers, distributors, or online platforms. Create agreements that will benefit both parties to maximize product distribution and sales channels.

3. Research Collaborations: Join forces with academic institutions or research centers to carry out research and development (R&D) for cutting-edge agricultural methods or aloe vera products. To remain competitive, make use of their resources and experience.

4. Form strategic alliances with businesses that complement each other in relevant industries, such as organic farming, health supplements, or natural skincare. Cross-promotional campaigns

and collaborative marketing can increase revenue and brand awareness.

5. Community Engagement: To promote social responsibility programs, sustainable farming methods, and community development projects, form alliances with nearby communities, non-governmental organizations, or environmental groups.

You may use the combined knowledge, assets, and networks of your strong partnerships and collaborations to further business expansion and make a good influence.

Long-Term Growth and Sustainability

Your aloe vera business needs to grow and sustain itself over the long term to succeed. Here are some crucial tactics to concentrate on:

1. Adopt sustainable agricultural techniques, such as managing soil health, conserving water, growing organic crops, and protecting

biodiversity. Make environmental stewardship a top priority to guarantee long-term viability.

2. Throughout the production process, maintain strict quality control methods to ensure the efficacy, safety, and quality of the final product. Invest in testing, certifications, and adherence to industry norms.

3. Brand Building: Invest in branding initiatives to set your aloe vera products apart from competitors. Create a compelling brand identity, share your beliefs with the world, and use marketing and storytelling to connect with consumers.

4. Continuous Innovation: To continuously improve your company's goods, procedures, and services, cultivate an innovative culture. Keep up with changes in technology, consumer tastes, and industry trends.

5. Customer satisfaction: Pay close attention to providing outstanding customer experiences by responding to comments from customers, adding value to products, and offering first-rate service. Increase advocacy and fidelity among your clientele.

6. Financial Management: Manage your money wisely by keeping an eye on expenses, allocating resources as efficiently as possible, and varying your sources of income. Remain financially resilient to handle market swings and economic difficulties.

It is possible to position your aloe vera firm for long-term sustainability, profitability, and growth by incorporating these techniques into your daily operations.